C000147332

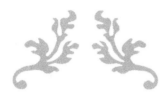

Low-Carb Cookbook for Beginners

Try Quick Easy and Delicious Low-Carb Recipes and
Discover How to Burn Stubborn Fat and Reset Metabolism
in 1 Week

Albert Lee

© Copyright 2021 - All rights reserved.

The content contained within this book may not be reproduced, duplicated or transmitted without direct written permission from the author or the publisher.

Under no circumstances will any blame or legal responsibility be held against the publisher, or author, for any damages, reparation, or monetary loss due to the information contained within this book. Either directly or indirectly.

Legal Notice:

This book is copyright protected. This book is only for personal use. You cannot amend, distribute, sell, use, quote or paraphrase any part, or the content within this book, without the consent of the author or publisher.

Disclaimer Notice:

Please note the information contained within this document is for educational and entertainment purposes only. All effort has been executed to present accurate, up to date, and reliable, complete information. No warranties of any kind are declared or implied. Readers acknowledge that the author is not engaging in the rendering of legal, financial, medical or professional advice. The content within this book has been derived from various sources. Please consult a licensed professional before attempting any techniques outlined in this book.

By reading this document, the reader agrees that under no circumstances is the author responsible for any losses, direct or indirect, which are incurred as a result of the use of information contained within this document, including, but not limited to, errors, omissions, or inaccuracies.

Table of Contents

1. Sweet And Savory Grilled Chicken 9
2. The Perfect Mediterranean Turkey Cutlets 11
3. Burnt Fried Chicken 13
4. Crunched Up Chicken Taco Wings 15
5. Tarragon Creamy Chicken 17
6. Spicy And Sour Chicken Breast 19
7. Spicy Grilled Chicken 21
8. Michigan Turkey Meal 23
9. Bacon Wrapped Chicken Breast With Spinach 25
10. Asparagus And Lemon Salmon Dish 27
11. Walnut Encrusted Salmon 29
12. Especial Glazed Salmon 31
13. Lovely Molten Tuna Bites 33
14. Hearty Lemon And Butter Cod 35
15. A Broccoli And Tilapia Dish To Die For! 37
16. Healthy Tuna Croquettes 39
17. Generous Stuffed Salmon Avocado 41
18. Baked Halibut Delight 43
19. Hungry Tuna Bites 45
20. Tilapia Broccoli Platter 47
21. Simple Baked Shrimp With Béchamel Sauce 49
22. Simple Sautéed Garlic And Parsley Scallops 51
23. Mesmerizing Coconut Haddock 53
24. "Salmon" Platter 55

25. Feisty Bacon Scallops 57

26. Grilled Lime Shrimp 59

27. Mouthwatering Calamari 61

28. Salmon And Zesty Cream Sauce 63

29. Crisped Up Coconut Shrimp 65

30. Spiced Up Tuna Avocado Balls 67

31. Asian Glazed Salmon and Cauliflower 69

32. Shrimp And Bacon Zoodles 71

33. Baked Lobster Tails And Garlic Butter 73

34. Spicy Sea Bass Hazelnuts 75

35. Perfectly Marinated Grilled Salmon 77

36. Salmon Fat Bombs 79

37. Baked Cod And Tomato Capers Delight 81

38. Perfect Tuna Salad And Pickle Boats 83

39. Tuna And Spinach Salad 85

40. Grilled Fish Salad Nicoise 87

41. Cumin And Salmon Meal 89

42. Favorite Lemon Dill Trout 91

43. Premium Dijon Halibut Steak 93

44. Asparagus And Tilapia Dish 95

45. Mesmerizing Shrimp Scampi 97

46. The All Time Favorite Tomato And Basil Soup 99

47. Healthy Lamb Stew 101

48. Hearty Chicken Liver Stew 103

49. Tender Slow Cooked Ham Stew 105

50.   Loving Cauliflower Soup 107

1. Sweet And Savory Grilled Chicken

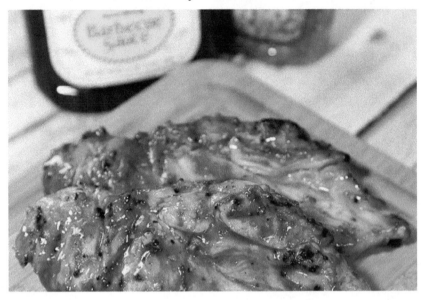

Serving: 4

Prep Time: 10 minutes

Cook Time: 12-15 minutes

<u>Ingredients</u>

- 1 teaspoon dry mustard
- 1 teaspoon light brown sugar
- 1 and 1/2 teaspoon onion powder
- 3/4 pound skinless chicken breast
- Kosher salt & White pepper

How To

1. Set the grill to preheat at medium-high temperatures as you add some greasing
2. In a small bowl, add onion powder, dry mustard, salt, brown sugar, and white pepper and mix well
3. Pass the chicken meat through the mixture to coat evenly.
4. Grill the chicken for 6 minutes on each side
5. Serve!

Nutrition (Per Serving)

- Calories: 176
- Fat: 4g
- Carbohydrates: 2g
- Protein: 30g

2. The Perfect Mediterranean Turkey Cutlets

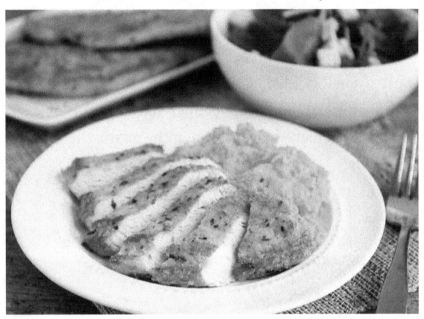

Serving: 4

Prep Time: 10 minutes

Cook Time: 12-15 minutes

Ingredients

- 1 tablespoon olive oil
- *1 and ¹/2 pound*turkey cutlets
- ¹/4 cup low carb flour mix
- ¹/2 teaspoon Greek seasoning
- ¹/2 teaspoon turmeric powder

How To

1. In a medium bowl, mix the turkey cutlets with turmeric powder, low carb flour mix, and Greek seasoning
2. Put a frying pan on fire, then add the oil to heat.
3. Add the cutlets and cook for 5 minutes on each side under medium-low heat.
4. Serve!

Nutrition (Per Serving)

- Calories: 283
- Fat: 13g
- Carbohydrates: 5g
- Protein: 34g

3. Burnt Fried Chicken

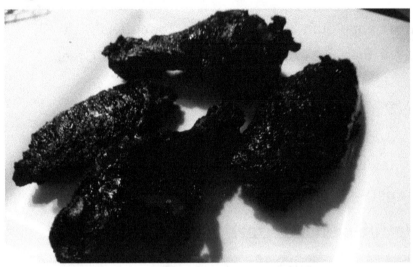

Serving: 4

Prep Time: 10 minutes

Cook Time: 20 minutes

Ingredients

- ¹/2 teaspoon cayenne pepper
- ¹/2 teaspoon onion powder
- ¹/2 teaspoon black pepper
- 2 teaspoons paprika
- 1 teaspoon ground thyme
- 1 teaspoon cumin
- ¹/4 teaspoon salt

- 2 (12-ounce / 340-g) skinless, boneless chicken breasts
- 2 teaspoons olive oil

How To

1. Mix the cayenne pepper, onion powder, black pepper, paprika, thyme, cumin, and salt in a bowl.

2. Rub the chicken breasts with the olive oil, then put it in the spice mixture. Make sure they are coated all around with the spices, then set aside to marinate for 5 minutes.

3. Preheat the air fryer to 375°F (190°C).

4. Put the chicken in the air fryer basket and cook for 10 minutes. Flip it over and cook for another 10 minutes.

5. Remove the chicken from the basket to a plate and let it rest for 5 minutes before serving.

Nutrition (Per Serving)

- Calories: 464
- Fat: 14g
- Carbohydrates: 3g
- Protein: 77g

4. Crunched Up Chicken Taco Wings

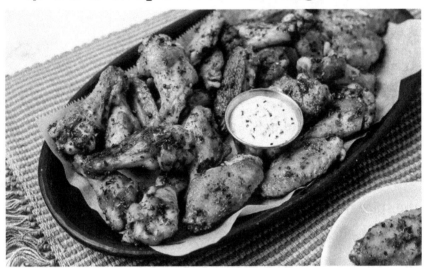

Serving: 4

Prep Time: 10 minutes

Cook Time: 15 minutes

Ingredients

- 3 pounds (1.4 kg) chicken wings
- 1 tablespoon taco seasoning mix
- 2 teaspoons olive oil

How To

1. Put the chicken wings in a Ziploc bag, then add the taco seasoning and olive oil.

2. Seal the bag and shake well until the chicken is coated thoroughly.

3. Preheat the air fryer to 350°F (180°C).

4. Put the chicken in the air fryer basket and cook for 6 minutes on each side until crispy.

5. Remove the chicken from the basket and serve on a plate.

<u>Nutrition (Per Serving)</u>

- Calories: 364
- Fat: 11g
- Carbohydrates: 1g
- Protein: 59g

5. Tarragon Creamy Chicken

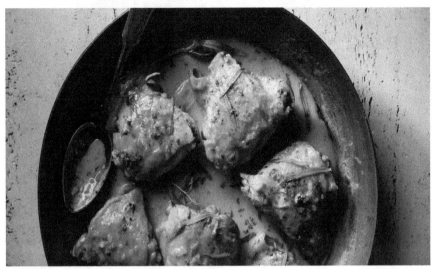

Serving: 4

Prep Time: 10 minutes

Cook Time: 30 minutes

Ingredients

- 1 tablespoon butter
- 1 tablespoon olive oil
- 4 skinless, boneless chicken breasts
- Salt and fleshly ground black pepper, to taste 1/2 cup heavy cream
- 1 tablespoon Dijon mustard
- 2 teaspoons chopped fresh tarragon

How To

1. Melt the butter in a pan over medium-high heat, then add the olive oil.

2. Season the chicken with salt and pepper then put it in the pan to fry for 15 minutes on both sides until the juices are clear. Remove them from the pan and set aside.

3. Pour the heavy cream in the pan and use a wooden spoon to scrape the parts stuck to the pan, then add the mustard and the tarragon. Mix well and let it simmer for 5 minutes.

4. Put the chicken back into the pan and cover it with the creamy sauce.

5. Serve the chicken drizzled with the sauce on a plate.

Nutrition (Per Serving)

- Calories: 400
- Fat: 18g
- Carbohydrates: 2g
- Protein: 53g

6. Spicy And Sour Chicken Breast

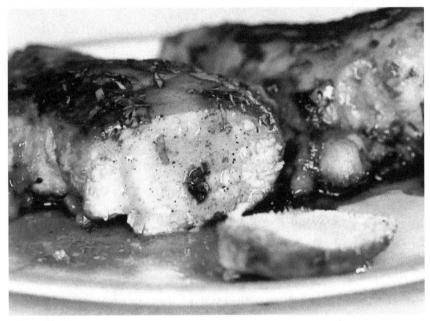

Serving: 4

Prep Time: 10 minutes

Cook Time: 10 minutes

Ingredients

- 4 skinless, boneless chicken breast halves 1/8 cup extra virgin olive oil
- 1 lemon, juiced
- 2 teaspoons crushed garlic
- 1 teaspoon salt
- 1 1/2 teaspoons black pepper

- ¹/3 teaspoon paprika
- 2 tablespoons olive oil, divided

How To

1. Combine the olive oil, lemon, garlic, salt, pepper, and paprika in a bowl, then set aside.

2. Cut 3 slits into the chicken breasts to allow the marinade to soak in. Put the chicken in a separate bowl and pour the marinade over it.

3. Cover the bowl with plastic wrap and put in the refrigerator to marinate overnight.

4. Preheat the grill to medium heat and brush the grill grates with 1 tablespoon of olive oil.

5. Remove the chicken from the marinade and place it on the grill to cook for about 5 minutes until the juices are clear. Flip the chicken over and brush with the remaining olive oil. Grill for 3 minutes more.

6. Remove the chicken from the grill and serve on plates.

Nutrition (Per Serving)

- Calories: 400
- Fat: 20g
- Carbohydrates: 2g
- Protein: 53g

7. Spicy Grilled Chicken

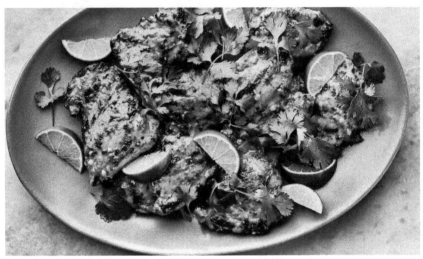

Serving: 4

Prep Time: 10 minutes

Cook Time: 20 minutes

Ingredients

- 1 teaspoon garlic powder
- 1 teaspoon ground paprika
- 1 teaspoon poultry seasoning
- 1 cup of olive oil
- *1/2 cup* apple cider vinegar
- 1 tablespoon salt
- 1 teaspoon black pepper
- 10 skinless chicken thighs

How To

1. Pour the garlic powder, paprika, poultry seasoning, oil, vinegar, salt, and black pepper into a jar with a lid, cover the jar and shake it well to combine.

2. Put the chicken thighs on a baking dish and pour three-quarters of the powder mixture over them. Cover the dish with plastic wrap and put it in the refrigerator to marinate for 8 hours, preferably overnight.

3. Preheat the grill to high heat.

4. Place the chicken on the grill to cook for 10 minutes on each side.

5. Transfer the chicken to a plate and brush with the remaining powder mixture, then serve.

Nutrition (Per Serving)

- Calories: 615
- Fat: 53g
- Carbohydrates: 1.2g
- Protein: 32g

8. Michigan Turkey Meal

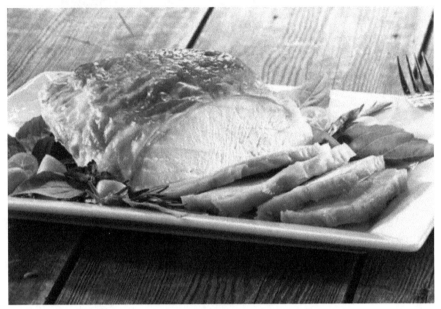

Serving: 4

Prep Time: 10 minutes

Cook Time: 4 Hours

Ingredients

- 1 (12-pound / 5.4-kg) whole turkey
- 6 tablespoons butter, divided
- 3 tablespoons chicken broth
- 4 cups warm water
- 2 tablespoons dried onion, minced
- 2 tablespoons dried parsley

- 2 tablespoons seasoning salt

How To

1. Start by preheating the oven to 350 °F (180 °C).

2. Rinse the turkey and pat dry with paper towels.

3. Put the turkey on a roasting pan, then separate the skin over the breast to make pockets.

4. Put 3 tablespoons of butter into each pocket.

5. Mix the broth and water in a medium bowl.

6. Add the minced onion and parsley, then pour over the turkey. Sprinkle some salt on the turkey then cover with aluminum foil.

7. Bake in the preheated oven until the internal temperatures of the turkey reads 180°F (80 °C), for about 4 hours.

8. When 45 minutes are remaining, remove the foil so that the turkey browns well.

9. Remove from the oven and serve warm.

Nutrition (Per Serving)

- Calories: 500
- Fat: 22g
- Carbohydrates: 0.6g
- Protein: 73g

9. Bacon Wrapped Chicken Breast With Spinach

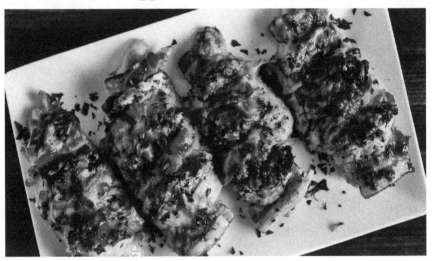

Serving: 4

Prep Time: 10 minutes

Cook Time: 10 minutes

Ingredients

- 1 (10-ounce / 284-g) package frozen chopped spinach, thawed and drained
- 1/2 cup mayonnaise, keto-friendly
- 1/2 cup feta cheese, shredded
- 2 cloves garlic, chopped
- 4 skinless, boneless chicken breasts 4 slices bacon

How To

1. Preheat the oven to 375²F (190²C).

2. Combine the spinach, mayo, feta cheese, and garlic in a bowl, then set aside.

3. Cut the chicken crosswise to butterfly the chicken breasts, (butterfly cutting technique: not to cut the chicken breast through, leave a 1-inch space uncut at the end of the chicken. So when flipping open the halved chicken breast, it resembles a butterfly.)

4. Unfold the chicken breasts like a book. Divide and arrange the spinach mixture over each breast, then wrap each breast with a slice of bacon and secure with a toothpick.

5. Arrange them in a baking dish, and cover a piece of aluminum foil. Place the dish in the preheated oven and bake for 1 hour or until the bacon is crispy and the juice of chicken breasts run clear.

6. Remove the baking dish from the oven and serve warm.

Nutrition (Per Serving)

- Calories: 626
- Fat: 41g
- Carbohydrates: 3.7g
- Protein: 61g

10.   Asparagus And Lemon Salmon Dish

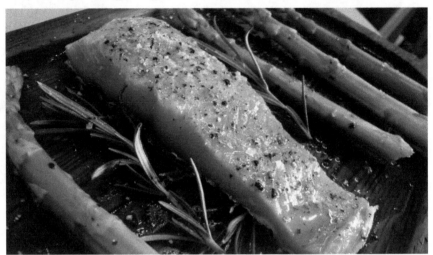

Serving: 3

Prep Time: 5 minutes

Cook Time: 15 minutes

Ingredients

- 2 salmon fillets, 6 ounces each, skin on
- Salt to taste
- 1 pound asparagus, trimmed
- 2 cloves garlic, minced
- 3 tablespoons butter
- ¼ cup parmesan cheese, grated

How To

1. Pre-heat your oven to 400 degree F

2. Line a baking sheet with oil

3. Take a kitchen towel and pat your salmon dry, season as needed

4. Put salmon around baking sheet and arrange asparagus around it

5. Place a pan over medium heat and melt butter

6. Add garlic and cook for 3 minutes until garlic browns slightly

7. Drizzle sauce over salmon

8. Sprinkle salmon with parmesan and bake for 12 minutes until salmon looks cooked all the way and is flaky

9. Serve and enjoy!

Nutrition (Per Serving)

- Calories: 434
- Fat: 26g
- Carbohydrates: 6g
- Protein: 42g

11. Walnut Encrusted Salmon

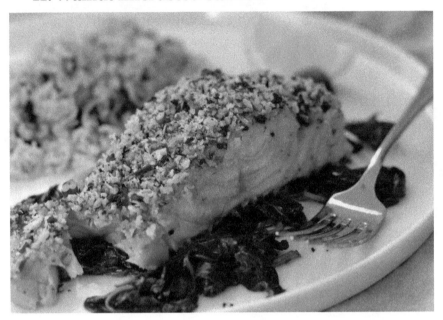

Serving: 3

Prep Time: 10 minutes

Cook Time: 14 minutes

<u>Ingredients</u>

- ½ cup walnuts
- 2 tablespoons stevia
- ½ tablespoon Dijon mustard
- ¼ teaspoon dill
- 2 Salmon fillets (3 ounces each)
- 1 tablespoon olive oil

- Salt and pepper to taste

How To

1. Pre-heat your oven to 350 degree F

2. Add walnuts, mustard, stevia to food processor and process until your desired consistency is achieved

3. Take a frying pan and place it over medium heat

4. Add oil and let it heat up

5. Add salmon and sear for 3 minutes

6. Add walnut mix and coat well

7. Transfer coated salmon to baking sheet, bake in oven for 8 minutes

8. Serve and enjoy!

Nutrition (Per Serving)

- Calories: 373
- Fat: 43g
- Carbohydrates: 4g
- Protein: 20g

12. Especial Glazed Salmon

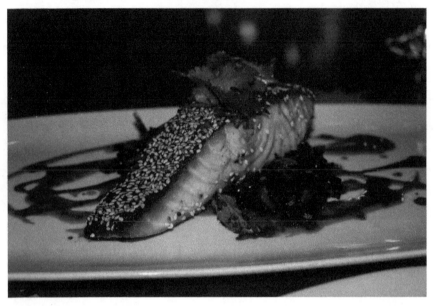

Serving: 4

Prep Time: 45 minutes

Cook Time: 10 minutes

Ingredients

- 4 pieces salmon fillets, 5 ounces each
- 4 tablespoons coconut aminos
- 4 teaspoon olive oil
- 2 teaspoon ginger, minced
- 4 teaspoon garlic, minced
- 2 tablespoon sugar-free ketchup
- 4 tablespoons dry white wine

31

- 2 tablespoons red boat fish sauce

How To

1. Take a bowl and mix in coconut aminos, garlic, ginger, fish sauce and mix

2. Add salmon and let it marinate for 15-20 minutes

3. Take a skillet/pan and place it over medium heat

4. Add oil and let it heat up

5. Add salmon fillets and cook on HIGH for 3-4 minutes per side

6. Remove dish once crispy

7. Add sauce and wine

8. Simmer for 5 minutes on low heat

9. Return salmon to the glaze and flip until both sides are glazed

10. Serve and enjoy!

Nutrition (Per Serving)

- Calories: 372
- Fat: 24g
- Carbohydrates: 3g
- Protein: 35g

13. Lovely Molten Tuna Bites

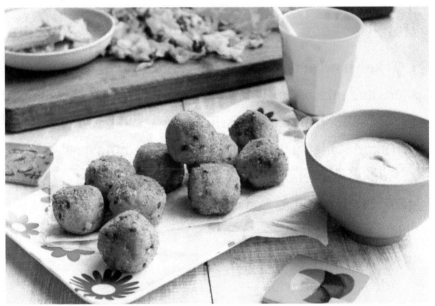

Serving: 4

Prep Time: 10 minutes

Cook Time: 10 minutes

Ingredients

- 10 ounces drained tuna
- ½ cup Keto-Friendly mayonnaise
- 1 medium avocado, cubed
- ¼ cup parmesan cheese
- ¼ cup almond flour
- ½ teaspoon garlic powder

33

- ¼ teaspoon onion powder
- Salt and pepper to taste
- ½ cup coconut oil

How To

1. Add the listed ingredients (except coconut oil) and avocado to a bowl and mix well

2. Take cubed avocado and fold them into tuna

3. Form balls from the mixture and dredge them in almond flour

4. Take a pan and place it over medium heat, add oil and let it heat up

5. Add tuna balls and fry until brown

6. Serve hot!

Nutrition (Per Serving)

- Calories: 134
- Fat: 11g
- Carbohydrates: 2g
- Protein: 7g

14. Hearty Lemon And Butter Cod

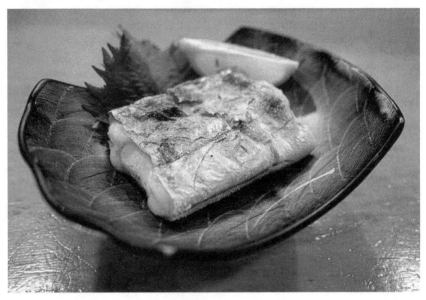

Serving: 3

Prep Time: 5 minutes

Cook Time: 20 minutes

Ingredients

- 4 tablespoons salted butter, divided
- 4 thyme sprigs, fresh and divided
- 4 teaspoons lemon juice, fresh and divided
- 4 cod fillets, 6 ounces each
- Salt to taste

How To

1. Pre-heat your oven to 400 degree F

2. Season cod fillets with salt on both side

3. Take four pieces of foil, each foil should be 3 times bigger than fillets

4. Divide fillets between the foils and top with butter, lemon juice, thyme

5. Fold to form a pouch and transfer pouches to baking sheet

6. Bake for 20 minutes

7. Open and let the steam get out

8. Serve and enjoy!

Nutrition (Per Serving)

- Calories: 284
- Fat: 18g
- Carbohydrates: 1g
- Protein: 32g

15. A Broccoli And Tilapia Dish To Die For!

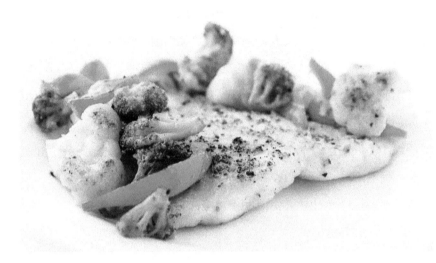

Serving: 1

Prep Time: 4 minutes

Cook Time: 14 minutes

Ingredients

- 6 ounce of tilapia, frozen
- 1 tablespoon of butter
- 1 tablespoon of garlic, minced
- 1 teaspoon of lemon pepper seasoning
- 1 cup of broccoli florets, fresh

How To

1. Pre-heat your oven to 350 degree Fahrenheit
2. Add fish in aluminum foil packets
3. Arrange broccoli around fish
4. Sprinkle lemon pepper on top
5. Close the packets and seal
6. Bake for 14 minutes
7. Take a bowl and add garlic and butter, mix well and keep the mixture on the side
8. Remove the packet from oven and transfer to platter
9. Place butter on top of the fish and broccoli, serve and enjoy!

Nutrition (Per Serving)

- Calories: 362
- Fat: 25g
- Net Carbohydrates: 2g
- Protein: 29g

16. Healthy Tuna Croquettes

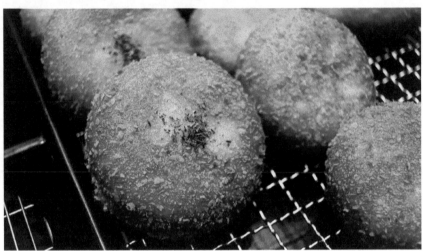

Serving: 4

Prep Time: 4 minutes

Cook Time: 9 minutes

Ingredients

- 1 can tuna, drained
- 1 whole large egg
- 8 tablespoons parmesan cheese, grated
- 2 tablespoons flax meal
- Salt and pepper to taste
- 1 tablespoons onion, minced

How To

1. Add all of the ingredients to a blender (except flax meal) and pulse them mixture into a crunchy texture

2. Form patties using the mixture

3. Dip both sides of the patties in flax meals and fry them in hot oil until both sides are browned well

Nutrition (Per Serving)

- Calories: 105
- Fat: 5g
- Carbohydrates: 2g
- Protein: 14g

17. Generous Stuffed Salmon Avocado

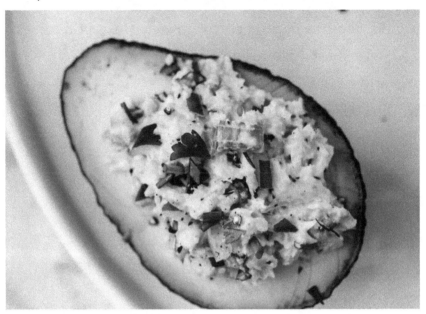

Serving: 2

Prep Time: 10 minutes

Cook Time: 30 minutes

Ingredients

- 1 ripe oragnic avocado
- 2 ounces wild caught smoked salmon
- 1 ounce fresh goat cheese
- 2 tablespoons extra virgin olive oil
- Salt as needed

How To

1. Cut avocado in half and deseed

2. Add rest of the ingredients to a food processor and process until coarsely chopped

3. Place mixture into avocado

4. Serve and enjoy!

Nutrition (Per Serving)

- Calories: 525
- Fat: 48g
- Carbohydrates: 4g
- Protein: 19g

18.Baked Halibut Delight

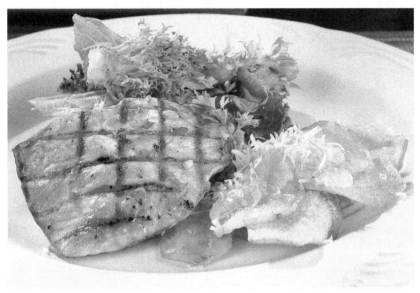

Serving: 8

Prep Time: 15 minutes

Cook Time: 30 minute

Ingredients

- 6 ounces halibut fillets
- 1 tablespoon Greek seasoning
- 1 large tomato, chopped
- 1 onion, chopped
- 5 ounces kalamata olives, pitted
- ¼ cup capers
- ¼ cup olive oil

- 1 tablespoon lemon juice
- Salt and pepper as needed

How To

1. Pre-heat your oven to 350 degree Fahrenheit
2. Transfer the halibut fillets on a large aluminum foil
3. Season with Greek seasoning
4. Take a bowl and add tomato, onion, olives, olive oil, capers, pepper, lemon juice and salt
5. Mix well and spoon the tomato mix over the halibut
6. Seal the edges and fold to make a packet
7. Place the packet on a baking sheet and bake in your oven for 30-40 minutes
8. Serve once the fish flakes off and enjoy!

Nutrition (Per Serving)

- Calories: 429
- Fat: 26g
- Carbohydrates: 10g
- Protein:36g

19. Hungry Tuna Bites

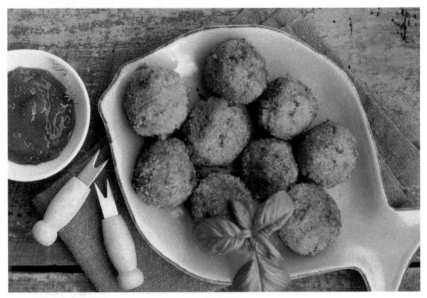

Serving: 2

Prep Time: 10 minutes

Cook Time: 10 minutes

Ingredients

- 10 ounces Canned Tuna, drained
- ¼ cup Keto Friendly mayonnaise
- 1 medium avocado, cubed
- ¼ cup parmesan cheese
- 1/3 cup almond flour
- ½ teaspoon garlic powder
- ¼ teaspoon onion powder

- Salt and pepper as needed
- ½ cup coconut oil

How To

1. Take a mixing bowl and add the listed ingredients except coconut oil and avocado

2. Take the cubed avocado and carefully fold them in the tuna mix

3. Mix well and turn the mixture into balls

4. Roll the balls into almond flour

5. Take a pan over medium heat and add coconut oil

6. Allow the oil to heat up

7. Add tuna balls and cook them well until you have a brown texture

8. Serve and enjoy!

Nutrition (Per Serving)

- Calories: 134
- Fat: 11g
- Carbohydrates: 2g
- Protein: 7g

20. Tilapia Broccoli Platter

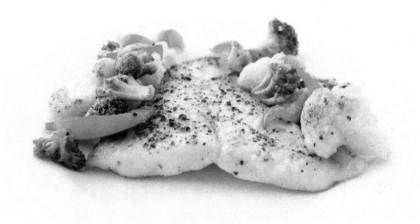

Serving: 2

Prep Time: 4 minutes

Cook Time: 14 minutes

Ingredients

- 6 ounce of tilapia, frozen
- 1 tablespoon of butter
- 1 tablespoon of garlic, minced
- 1 teaspoon of lemon pepper seasoning
- 1 cup of broccoli florets, fresh

How To

1. Pre-heat your oven to 350 degree F
2. Add fish in aluminum foil packets

3. Arrange broccoli around fish

4. Sprinkle lemon pepper on top

5. Close the packets and seal

6. Bake for 14 minutes

7. Take a bowl and add garlic and butter, mix well and keep the mixture on the side

8. Remove the packet from oven and transfer to platter

9. Place butter on top of the fish and broccoli, serve and enjoy!

Nutrition (Per Serving)

- Calories: 362
- Fat: 25g
- Carbohydrates: 2g
- Protein: 29g

21. Simple Baked Shrimp With Béchamel Sauce

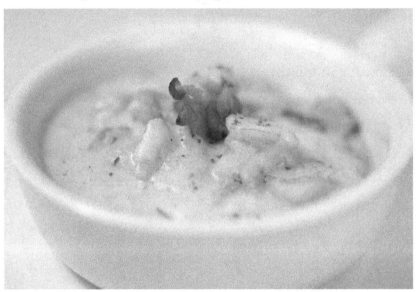

Serving: 4

Prep Time: 10 minutes

Cook Time: 5-7 minutes

Ingredients

- 6-7 ounces shrimp
- 1 ounce mozzarella
- 4 ounces béchamel sauce (recipe provided)
- 1 tablespoons ghee

How To

1. Cut boiled shrimp and transfer them to baking dish

2. Pour sauce on top

3. Bake for 5-7 minutes

4. Serve and enjoy!

<u>Nutrition (Per Serving)</u>

- Calories: 150
- Fat: 10g
- Carbohydrates: 2g
- Protein: 14g

22.   Simple Sautéed Garlic And Parsley Scallops

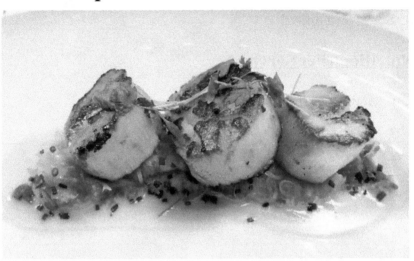

Serving: 4

Prep Time: 5 minutes

Cook Time: 25 minutes

Ingredients

- 8 tablespoons butter
- 2 garlic cloves, minced
- 16 large sea scallops
- Salt and pepper to taste
- 1 and ½ tablespoons olive oil

How To

1. Seasons scallops with salt and pepper

2. Take a skillet and place it over medium heat, add oil and let it heat up

3. Saute scallops for 2 minutes per side, repeat until all Scallops are cooked

4. Add butter to the skillet and let it melt

5. Stir in garlic and cook for 15 minutes

6. Return scallops to skillet and stir to coat

7. Serve and enjoy!

Nutrition (Per Serving)

- Calories: 417
- Fat: 31g
- Net Carbohydrates: 5g
- Protein: 29g

23.   Mesmerizing Coconut Haddock

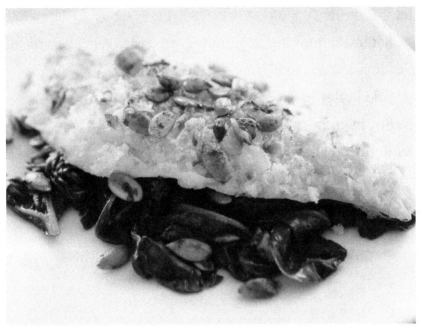

Serving: 3

Prep Time: 10 minutes

Cook Time: 12 minutes

Ingredients

- 4 haddock fillets, 5 ounces each, boneless
- 2 tablespoons coconut oil, melted
- 1 cup coconut, shredded and unsweetened
- ¼ cup hazelnuts, ground
- Salt to taste

How To

1. Pre-heat your oven to 400-degree F

2. Line a baking sheet with parchment paper

3. Keep it on the side

4. Pat fish fillets with paper towel and season with salt

5. Take a bowl and stir in hazelnuts and shredded coconut

6. Drag fish fillets through the coconut mix until both sides are coated well

7. Transfer to baking dish

8. Brush with coconut oil

9. Bake for about 12 minutes until flaky

10. Serve and enjoy!

Nutrition (Per Serving)

- Calories: 299
- Fat: 24g
- Carbohydrates: 1g
- Protein: 20g

24.   "Salmon" Platter

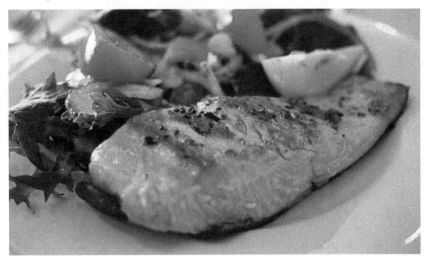

Serving: 3

Prep Time: 5 minute

Cook Time: 6 minutes

Ingredients

- ¾ cup of water
- Few sprigs of parsley, basil, tarragon, basil
- 1 pound of salmon , skin on
- 3 teaspoon of ghee
- ¼ teaspoon of salt
- ½ teaspoon of pepper
- ½ of a lemon, thinly sliced
- 1 whole carrot, julienned

How To

1. Set your pot to Saute mode and water and herbs

2. Place a steamer rack inside your pot and place salmon

3. Drizzle Ghee on top of the salmon and season with salt and pepper

4. Cover lemon slices

5. Lock up the lid and cook on HIGH pressure for 3 minutes

6. Release the pressure naturally over 10 minutes

7. Transfer the salmon to a serving platter

8. Set your pot to Saute mode and add vegetables

9. Cook for 1-2 minutes

10. Serve with vegetables and salmon

11. Enjoy!

Nutrition Values (Per Serving)

- Calories: 464
- Fat: 34g
- Carbohydrates: 3g
- Protein: 34g

25.   Feisty Bacon Scallops

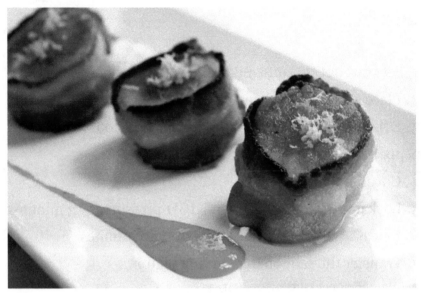

Serving: 4

Prep Time: 10 minutes

Cook Time: 23 minutes

Ingredients

- 1 pound bacon, uncured
- 2 pounds sea scallops, fresh and patted dry
- Lemon wedges
- 3 tablespoon golden ghee
- ¼ cup dry white wine

How To

1. Line two baking sheets with parchment paper

2. Pre-heat your oven to 400-degree F

3. Put bacon strips on sheet evenly, bake for 15 minutes

4. Crumbled once cooked and cooled

5. Take a skillet and place it over high heat

6. Pour grease and heat it up

7. Brown scallops in oil, cook for 3 minutes each side

8. Set scallops on the side and add wine to the skillet

9. Use wine to deglaze pan, scrape brown bits

10. Add ghee and make wine sauce

11. Add scallops and bacon

12. Toss and cook for 1 minute more

13. Enjoy!

Nutrition (Per Serving)

- Calories: 550
- Fat: 27g
- Carbohydrates: 6g
- Protein: 66g

26.   Grilled Lime Shrimp

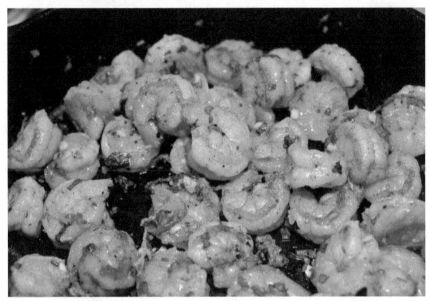

Serving: 8

Prep Time: 25 minutes

Cook Time: 5 minutes

Ingredients

- 1 pound medium shirmp, peeled and deveined
- 1 lime, juiced
- ½ cup olive oil
- 3 tablespoons Cajun seasoning

How To

1. Take a re-sealable zip bag and add lime juice, Cajun seasoning, olive oil

2. Add shrimp and shake it well, let it marinate for 20 minutes

3. Pre-heat your outdoor grill to medium heat

4. Lightly grease the grate

5. Remove shrimp from marinade and cook for 2 minutes per side

6. Serve and enjoy!

Nutrition (Per Serving)

- Calories: 188
- Fat: 3g
- Net Carbohydrates: 1.2g
- Protein: 13g

27.   Mouthwatering Calamari

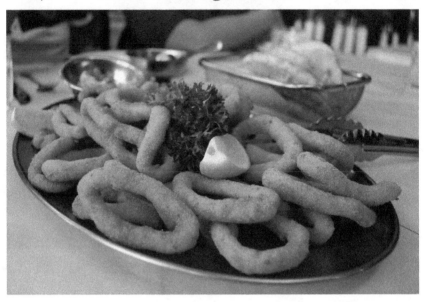

Serving: 4

Prep Time: 10 minutes +1-hour marinating

Cook Time: 8 minutes

Ingredients

- 2 tablespoons extra virgin olive oil
- 1 teaspoon chili powder
- ½ teaspoon ground cumin
- Zest of 1 lime
- Juice of 1 lime
- Dash of sea salt

- 1 and ½ pounds squid, cleaned and split open, with tentacles cut into ½ inch rounds
- 2 tablespoons cilantro, chopped
- 2 tablespoons red bell pepper, minced

How To

1. Take a medium bowl and stir in olive oil, chili powder, cumin, lime zest, sea salt, lime juice and pepper

2. Add squid and let it marinade and stir to coat, coat and let it refrigerate for 1 hour

3. Pre-heat your oven to broil

4. Arrange squid on a baking sheet, broil for 8 minutes turn once until tender

5. Garnish the broiled calamari with cilantro and red bell pepper

6. Serve and enjoy!

Nutrition (Per Serving)

- Calories: 159
- Fat: 13g
- Carbohydrates: 12g
- Protein: 3g

28.   Salmon And Zesty Cream Sauce

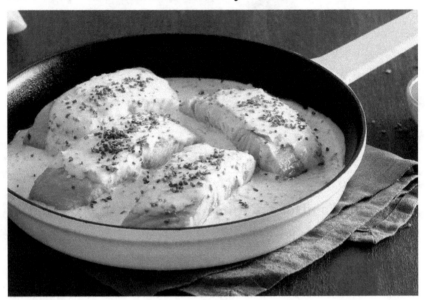

Serving: 4

Prep Time: 10 minutes

Cook Time: 5-7 minutes

Ingredients

- 2 boneless salmon or trout fillets
- 1/3 cup sour cream
- 2 tsp mustard
- 1 tbsp lemon juice
- 1/2 tsp dill
- 1 tsp lemon zest

How To

1. Mix all the cream ingredients and spices together in a small bowl.

2. Season with salt and pepper to taste and set aside.

3. Lightly grease a shallow pan and cook the fillets for 2-3 minutes on each side (for a medium to well-done result).

4. Serve on a dish and pour the sauce on top or on the side. You can serve it also with some broccoli or asparagus for an extra kick of taste and nutrients

Nutrition (Per Serving)

- Calories: 397
- Fat: 22g
- Carbohydrates: 4g
- Protein: 42g

29.   Crisped Up Coconut Shrimp

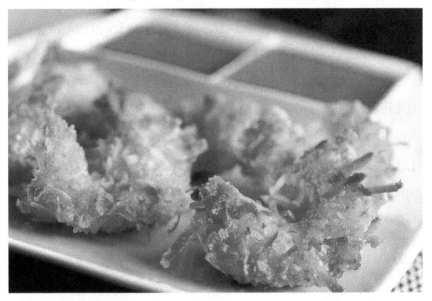

Serving: 4

Prep Time: 10 minutes

Cook Time: 20 minutes

<u>Ingredients</u>

- 1 pound of large shrimp (peeled and deveined)
- ½ cup coconut flour
- 1 tsp cayenne seasoning (salt included)
- 3 eggs beaten
- 1/2 cup unsweetened coconut flakes

How To

1. Keep the coconut flour with the seasoning, coconut flakes, and beaten eggs into separate bowls each.

2. Dip and roll in the shrimps (one by one) into the coconut flour mixture, shake off the excess flour, dip in the eggs and then roll in last to the unsweetened coconut flakes.

3. Heat one cup of oil and dry the shrimps for 4-5 minutes or until golden brown.

4. Serve in a shallow dish with absorbing paper and serve with hot mayo (mayo with cayenne seasoning)

Nutrition (Per Serving)

- Calories: 354
- Fat: 24g
- Carbohydrates: 20g
- Protein: 13g

30.   Spiced Up Tuna Avocado Balls

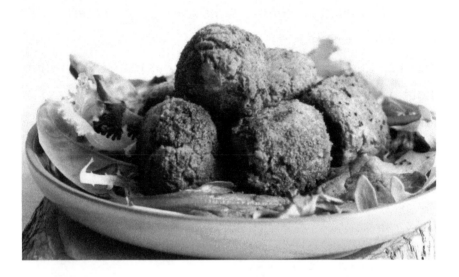

Serving: 4

Prep Time: 10 minutes

Cook Time: Nil

Ingredients

- 2 avocados halved
- 1/2 lbof sushi-grade ahi tuna (or smoked tuna if you can't find any)
- 2 tbsp of mayo
- 1-2 sriracha sauce
- 1 tsp of toasted sesame seeds

How To

1. Combine in a small bowl the tuna with the mayo, sriracha sauce, and toasted sesame seeds.

2. Scoop and distribute the mixture onto the avocado halves.

3. Add some extra sriracha sauce optionally on top

Nutrition (Per Serving)

- Calories: 256
- Fat: 17g
- Carbohydrates: 8g
- Protein: 15g

31. Asian Glazed Salmon and Cauliflower

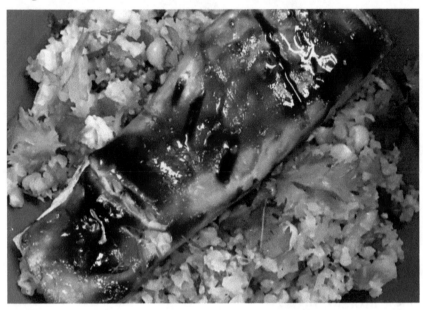

Serving: 4

Prep Time: 10 minutes

Cook Time: 5 minutes

Ingredients

- 4 boneless fillets of salmon
- 2 cups (around 550 grams) of frozen cauliflower rice (or freshly ground cauliflower rice using a food processor)
- 4 tbsp of liquid aminos or soy sauce
- 2 tbsp of shallots, chopped finely
- 2 tbsp of sesame oil

How To

1. Make a marinade of the liquid aminos, shallots, and sesame oil and combine them all into a bowl.

2. Soak the salmon fillets to the marinade and optionally refrigerate for at least an hour before cooking.

3. Pop these into the oven and bake for 10-12 minutes.

4. While the salmon cooks, heat and prepare the frozen cauliflower rice, according to package instructions.

5. Serve the salmon over the cauliflower rice hot

Nutrition (Per Serving)

- Calories: 210
- Fat: 13g
- Carbohydrates: 4g
- Protein: 15g

32. Shrimp And Bacon Zoodles

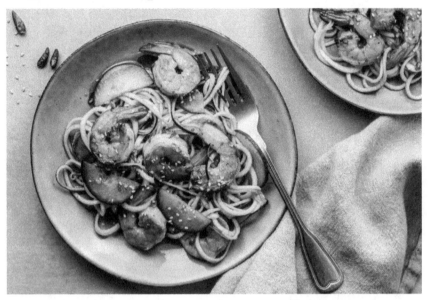

Serving: 4

Prep Time: 10 minutes

Cook Time: 12 minutes

<u>Ingredients</u>

- 1 lb of fresh peeled and deveined shrimp
- 5/4 cup of salted butter
- 2 cloves of garlic mashed
- 2-3 stripes of beef bacon, chopped
- 1 zucchini, made into zoodles using a spiralizer or mandolin slicer

How To

1. Heat a skillet, add the butter and shrimp and cook for 2 minutes on each side.

2. Add the garlic and cook for another minute.

3. Remove the shrimps from the heat and add the bacon and the zucchini noodles in the garlic oil. Cook tossing for 4-5 minutes.

4. Return the shrimps to the bacon zoodles, toss, and transfer to a deep dish.

5. Sprinkle optionally with some freshly grated parmesan

Nutrition (Per Serving)

- Calories: 670
- Fat: 51g
- Carbohydrates: 6g
- Protein: 48g

33. Baked Lobster Tails And Garlic Butter

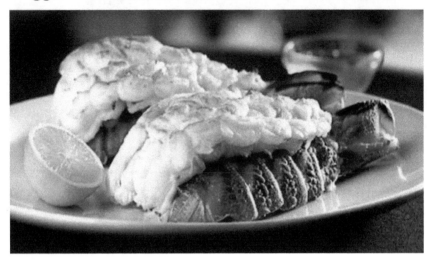

Serving: 4

Prep Time: 10 minutes

Cook Time: 15 minutes

Ingredients

- 4 lobster tails
- 1 lemon juiced
- 5 cloves of garlic
- 1/4 cup grated parmesan
- 4 tbsp of salted butter

How To

1. Preheat oven to 375F/180C. In a small bowl, combine together the lemon juice, garlic, and grated parmesan.

2. Using kitchen shears, cut the clear skin and remove off the lobster and brush the tails with the garlic butter mix.

3. Place on a baking sheet with parchment paper on top and bake in the oven for 15 minutes

Nutrition (Per Serving)

- Calories: 222
- Fat: 14g
- Carbohydrates: 2g
- Protein: 21g

34.   Spicy Sea Bass Hazelnuts

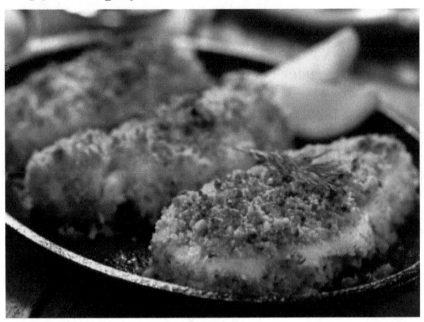

Serving: 4

Prep Time: 10 minutes

Cook Time: 15-20 minutes

Ingredients

- 2 sea bass fillets
- 2 tbsp butter
- 1/3 cup roasted hazelnuts
- A pinch of cayenne pepper

How To

1. Preheat your oven to 425⁵F.
2. Line a baking dish with waxed paper. Melt the butter and brush it over the fish.
3. Process the cayenne pepper and hazelnuts in a food processor to achieve a smooth consistency. Coat the sea bass with the hazelnut mixture.
4. Place in the oven and bake for about 15 minutes

Nutrition (Per Serving)

- Calories: 467
- Fat: 31g
- Carbohydrates: 3.8g
- Protein: g

35.   Perfectly Marinated Grilled Salmon

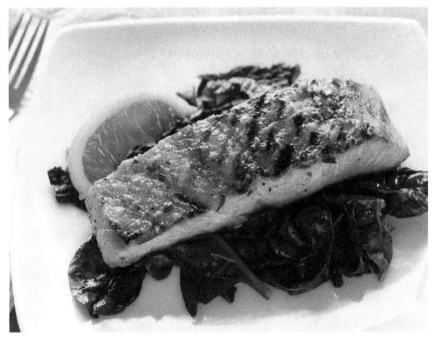

Serving: 4

Prep Time: 10-50 minutes

Cook Time: 10-20 minutes

Ingredients

- 4 5-ounce salmon steaks
- 2 cloves garlic, pressed
- 4 tablespoons olive oil
- 1 tablespoon Taco seasoning mix
- 2 tablespoons fresh lemon juice

How To

1. Place all of the above ingredients in a ceramic dish; cover and let it marinate for 40 minutes in your refrigerator.
2. Place the salmon steaks onto a lightly oiled grill pan; place under the grill for 6 minutes.
3. Turn them over and cook for a further 5 to 6 minutes, basting with the reserved marinade; remove from the grill.
4. Serve immediately and enjoy

Nutrition (Per Serving)

- Calories: 3312
- Fat: 2g
- Carbohydrates: 30g
- Protein: 0.4g

36. Salmon Fat Bombs

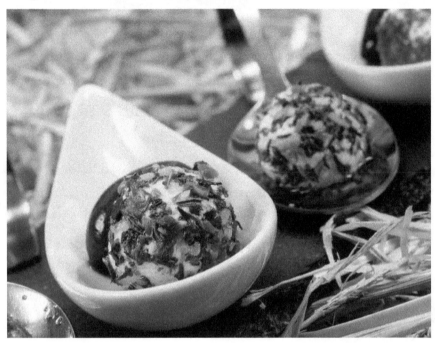

Serving: 4

Prep Time: 10 minutes

Cook Time: Nil

Ingredients

- 2 tbsp cream cheese, softened
- 1 ounce smoked salmon
- 2 tsp bagel seasoning

How To

1. Take a medium bowl, place cream cheese and salmon in it, and stir until well combined.

2. Shape the mixture into balls, roll them into bagel seasoning and then serve

Nutrition (Per Serving)

- Calories: 48
- Fat: 4g
- Carbohydrates: 0g
- Protein: 0..5g

Baked Cod And Tomato Capers Delight

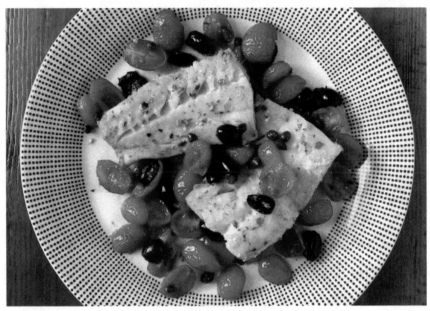

Serving: 4

Prep Time: 10 minutes

Cook Time: 25 minutes

Ingredients

- 4 cod fillets, boneless
- 2 tablespoons avocado oil
- 1 cup tomato passata
- 2 tablespoons capers, drained
- 2 tablespoons parsley, chopped

How To

1. In a roasting pan, combine the cod with the oil and the other ingredients, toss gently, introduce in the oven at 370 degrees F and bake for 25 minutes.

2. Divide between plates and serve

Nutrition (Per Serving)

- Calories: 150
- Fat: 3g
- Carbohydrates: 0.7g
- Protein: 3g

38.   Perfect Tuna Salad And Pickle Boats

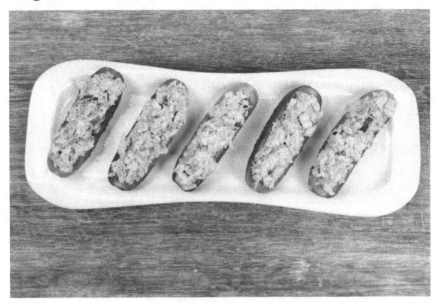

Serving: 4

Prep Time: 10 minutes + 30 minutes chill time

Cook Time: Nil

<u>Ingredients</u>

- 18 oz canned and drained tuna
- 6 large dill pickles
- ¹/a tsp garlic powder
- ¹/4 cup sugar-free mayonnaise
- 1 tsp onion powder

How To

1. Mix the mayo, tuna, onion, and garlic powders in a bowl. Cut the pickles in half, lengthwise. Top each half with a tuna mixture.

2. Place in the fridge for 30 minutes and serve

Nutrition (Per Serving)

- Calories: 118
- Fat: 10g
- Carbohydrates: 1.5g
- Protein: 11g

39.   Tuna And Spinach Salad

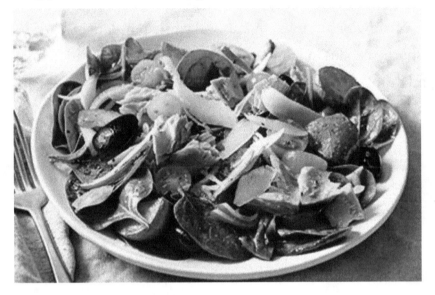

Serving: 4

Prep Time: 10 minutes

Cook Time: Nil

<u>Ingredients</u>

- 2 oz of spinach leaves
- 2 oz tuna, packed in water
- 1/4 tsp ground black pepper
- 1/4 tsp sea salt
- 2 tbsp coconut oil, melted

How To

1. Take a salad bowl, place spinach leaves in it, drizzle with 1 tbsp oil, sprinkle with 1/8 tsp of salt and black pepper, and then toss until mixed.

2. Top with tuna, sprinkle with remaining salt and black pepper, drizzle with oil and then serve

Nutrition (Per Serving)

- Calories: 155
- Fat: 62g
- Carbohydrates: 1.3g
- Protein: 0.7g

40.   Grilled Fish Salad Nicoise

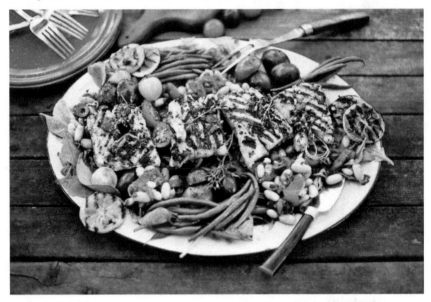

Serving: 4

Prep Time: 10 minutes

Cook Time: 10-15 minutes

Ingredients

- 3/4 pound tuna fillet, skinless
- 1 white onion, sliced
- 1 teaspoon Dijon mustard
- 8 Nicoise olives, pitted and sliced
- 1/2 teaspoon anchovy paste

How To

1. Brush the tuna with nonstick cooking oil; season with salt and freshly cracked black pepper. Then, grill your tuna on a lightly oiled rack for approximately 7 minutes, turning over once or twice.

2. Let the fish stand for 3 to 4 minutes and break into bite-sized pieces. Transfer to a nice salad bowl.

3. Toss the tuna pieces with the white onion, Dijon mustard, Nicoise olives, and anchovy paste. Serve well chilled, and enjoy!

Nutrition (Per Serving)

- Calories: 194
- Fat: 0.9g
- Carbohydrates: 3.7g
- Protein: 0.5g

41.Cumin And Salmon Meal

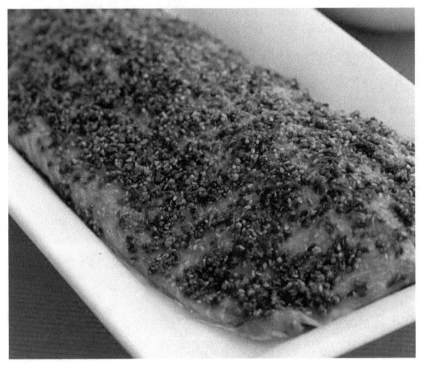

Serving: 4

Prep Time: 10 minutes

Cook Time: 2-5 minutes

Ingredients

- 4 salmon fillets, boneless
- 1 tablespoon avocado oil
- 1 red onion, sliced
- 1 teaspoon chili powder
- l teaspoon cumin, ground

How To

1. Heat up a pan with the oil over medium-high heat, add the onion and chili powder and cook for 2 minutes.
2. Add the fish, salt, pepper, and cumin, cook for 4 minutes on each side divide between plates and serve.

Nutrition (Per Serving)

- Calories: 300
- Fat: 14g
- Carbohydrates: 5g
- Protein: 20g

42.   Favorite Lemon Dill Trout

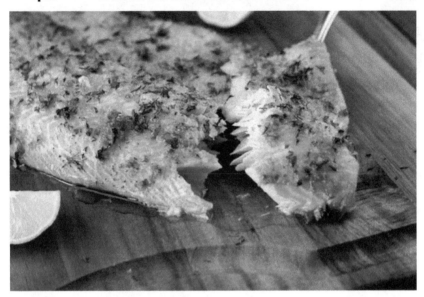

Serving: 4

Prep Time: 10 minutes

Cook Time: 5-10 minutes

Ingredients

- 2 lb pan-dressed trout (or other small fish), fresh or frozen
- 1 ¹12 tsp salt
- ¹/2 cup butter or margarine
- 2 tbsp dill weed
- 3 tbsp lemon juice

How To

1. Cut the fish lengthwise and season it with pepper.
2. Prepare a skillet by melting the butter and dill weed.
3. Fry the fish on high heat, flesh side down, for 2-3 minutes per side.
4. Remove the fish. Add the lemon juice to the butter and dill to create a sauce.
5. Serve the fish with the sauce.

Nutrition (Per Serving)

- Calories: 460
- Fat: 22g
- Carbohydrates: 1g
- Protein: 57g

43.   Premium Dijon Halibut Steak

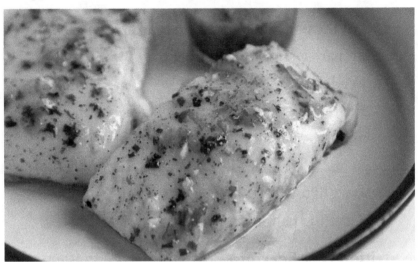

Serving: 4

Prep Time: 10 minutes

Cook Time: 10-20 minutes

Ingredients

- 1 6-oz fresh or thawed halibut steak
- 1 tbsp butter
- 1 tbsp lemon juice
- 1/2 tbsp Dijon mustard
- 1 tsp fresh basil

How To

1. Heat the butter, basil, lemon juice, and mustard in a small saucepan to make a glaze.
2. Brush both sides of the halibut steak with the mixture.
3. Grill the fish for 10 minutes over medium heat until tender and flakey.

Nutrition (Per Serving)

- Calories: 305
- Fat: 16g
- Carbohydrates: 6g
- Protein: 34g

44.   Asparagus And Tilapia Dish

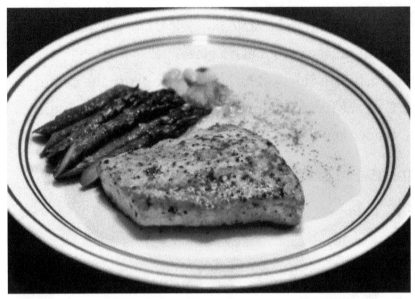

Serving: 4

Prep Time: 20 minutes

Cook Time:2 hours

<u>Ingredients</u>

- 1 bunch asparagus
- 4-6 tilapia fillets
- 8-12 tablespoons lemon juice
- Pepper for seasoning
- Lemon juice for seasoning
- ½ tablespoons for clarified butter, for each fillet

How To

1. Cut single pieces of foil for the fillets

2. Divide the bundle of asparagus into even number depending on the number of your fillets

3. Lay the fillets on each of the pieces of foil and sprinkle pepper and add a teaspoon of lemon juice

4. Add clarified butter and top with asparagus

5. Fold the foil over the fish and seal the ends

6. Repeat with all the fillets and transfer to cooker

7. Cook on HIGH for 2 hours

8. Enjoy!

Nutrition (Per Serving)

- Calories: 229
- Fat: 10g
- Carbohydrates: 1g
- Protein: 28g

45.   Mesmerizing Shrimp Scampi

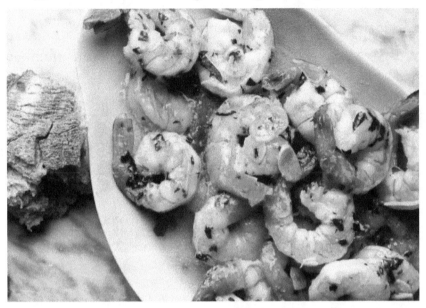

Serving: 3

Prep Time: 20 minutes

Cook Time:2 hours 30 minutes

Ingredients

- 1 cup chicken broth
- ½ cup white wine vinegar
- 2 tablespoons olive oil
- 2 teaspoon garlic, chopped
- 2 teaspoons garlic, minced
- 1 pound large raw shrimp

How To

1. Add chicken broth, lemon juice, white wine vinegar, olive oil, lemon juice, chopped garlic, and fresh minced parsley
2. Add thawed shrimp (the ratio should be 1 pound of shrimp for ¼ cup of chicken broth)
3. Place lid and cook on LOW for 2 and a ½ hours
4. Serve and enjoy!

Nutrition (Per Serving)

- Calories: 293
- Fat: 24g
- Carbohydrates: 4g
- Protein: 16g

46. The All Time Favorite Tomato And Basil Soup

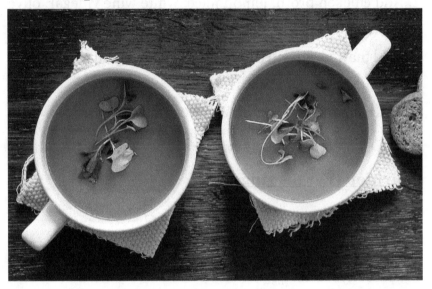

Serving: 4

Prep Time: 10 minutes

Cook Time: 15 minutes

Ingredients

- 14.5 ounces tomatoes, diced
- 2 ounces cream cheese
- ¼ cup heavy whipping cream
- ¼ cup basil, fresh and chopped
- 4 tablespoons butter

How To

1. Add tomatoes into blender, alongside juices and puree until smooth

2. Take a saucepan and place it over medium heat, add tomato puree, heavy cream, butter, cream cheese and cook for 10 minutes

3. Add basil, season as desired and cook for 5 minutes more

4. Use an immersion blender to blend the mixture

5. Serve and enjoy!

Nutrition (Per Serving)

- Calories: 239
- Fat: 22g
- Carbohydrates: 7g
- Protein: 3g

Healthy Lamb Stew

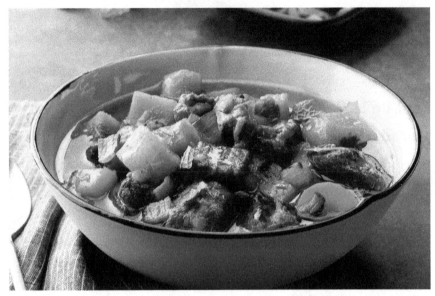

Serving: 4

Prep Time: 10 minutes

Cook Time: 3 hours

Ingredients

- 1 onion, peeled and chopped
- 3 carrots, peeled and chopped
- 2 pounds lamb, cubed
- 1 tomato, cored and chopped
- 1 garlic clove, peeled and minced
- 2 tablespoons butter
- 1 cup beef stock

- 1 cup white wine
- Salt and pepper to taste
- 2 rosemary sprigs
- 1 teaspoon fresh thyme, chopped

How To

1. Heat up Dutch oven over medium-high heat
2. Add oil and let it heat up
3. Add lamb, salt, pepper and brown all sides
4. Transfer to plate
5. Add onion to Dutch oven and cook for 2 minutes
6. Add carrots, tomato, garlic, butter stick, wine, salt, pepper, rosemary, thyem and stir for a few minutes
7. Return lamb to Dutch Oven and cook for4 hours
8. Discard rosemary sprits
9. Add more salt, pepper and stir
10. Divide between bowls
11. Serve and enjoy!

Nutrition (Per Serving)

- Calories: 700
- Fat: 43g
- Carbohydrates: 10g
- Protein: 67g

48.   Hearty Chicken Liver Stew

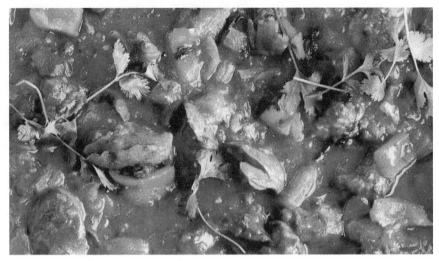

Serving: 2

Prep Time: 10 minutes

Cook Time: Nil

Ingredients

- 10 ounces chicken livers
- 1 ounce onion, chopped
- 2 ounces sour cream
- 1 tablespoon olive oil
- Salt to taste

How To

1. Take a pan and place it over medium heat

2. Add oil and let it heat up

3. Add onions and fry until just browned

4. Add livers and season with salt

5. Cook until livers are half cooked

6. Transfer the mix to a stew pot

7. Add sour cream and cook for 20 minutes

8. Serve and enjoy!

Nutrition (Per Serving)

- Calories: 146
- Fat: 9g
- Carbohydrates: 2g
- Protein: 15g

49.   Tender Slow Cooked Ham Stew

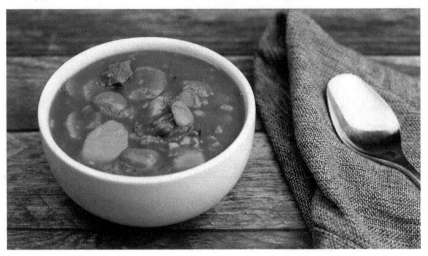

Serving: 4

Prep Time: 10 minutes

Cook Time: 4 hours

Ingredients

- 8 ounces cheddar cheese, grated
- 14 ounces chicken stock
- ½ teaspoon garlic powder
- Salt and pepper to taste
- 4 garlic cloves, peeled and minced
- ¼ cup heavy cream
- 3 cups ham, chopped
- 16 ounces cauliflower florets

- 1 cup carrot, sliced into thin rings

How To

1. Add ham, stock, cheese, cauliflower, garlic powder, onion powder, salt, pepper, garlic, carrot, heavy cream to Slow Cooker

2. Stir well

3. Place lid and cook on HIGH for 4 hours

4. Stir and divide between bowls

5. Serve and enjoy!

Nutrition (Per Serving)

- Calories: 320
- Fat: 20g
- Carbohydrates: 6g
- Protein: 23g

50.   Loving Cauliflower Soup

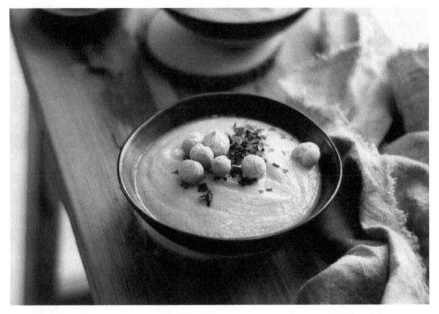

Serving: 6

Prep Time: 10 minutes

Cook Time: 10 minutes

<u>Ingredients</u>

- 4 cups vegetable stock
- 1 pound cauliflower, trimmed and chopped
- 7 ounces cream cheese
- 4 ounces butter
- Salt and pepper to taste

How To

1. Take a skillet and place it over medium heat

2. Add butter and melt

3. Add cauliflower and Saute for 2 minutes

4. Add stock and bring mix to a boil

5. Cook until Cauliflower are Al-Dente

6. Stir in cream cheese, salt and pepper

7. Puree the mix using immersion blender

8. Serve and enjoy!

Nutrition (Per Serving)

- Calories: 143
- Fat: 16g
- Carbohydrates: 6g
- Protein: 3.4g

CPSIA information can be obtained
at www.ICGtesting.com
Printed in the USA
BVHW051129260721
612866BV00010B/636